is essential.

In addition, this eBook emphasizes the importance of setting realistic and attainable goals. By breaking down larger goals into smaller, manageable tasks, we can foster a sense of progress and motivation that keeps us on track. We will also explore the vital role of support systems and how the encouragement of friends, family, and like-minded communities can significantly enhance our commitment and drive.

Central to our discussion is the topic of eating habits. Choosing to eat healthily is often perceived as a battle between immediate gratification and long-term health. We'll look at how emotional eating and societal pressures can warp our relationship with food, turning it into a source of guilt rather than nourishment. By adopting a view of food as essential fuel for our body and spirit, we can transform our eating habits into powerful tools for health improvement.

This eBook offers practical advice for navigating the complexities of making healthier food choices. From understanding the fundamentals of nutrition to recognizing our body's needs, we'll outline key strategies for making food a friend rather than a foe. Whether your goal is a complete diet overhaul or simply more mindful eating, the aim is to empower you to take control of your eating habits in a manner that supports your overall health and happiness.

Join us on this journey to sustainable eating habit changes, fostering a positive relationship with food, and ultimately leading a life that is not only healthier but more fulfilling. Welcome to the path of regulated eating strategies, where food becomes a cornerstone of a vibrant, energetic, and healthier you.

Terms and Conditions & Legal Disclaimer

The Publisher has dedicated considerable effort to ensure the accuracy and completeness of this report, fully aware that the dynamic and ever-evolving nature of the Internet means that the content may not always mirror the latest developments or insights. Despite meticulous attempts to verify all information presented in this publication, the Publisher acknowledges the possibility of inaccuracies or misinterpretations and, as such, cannot be held responsible for any errors, omissions, or misunderstandings within the text. It is not, and never has been, the intention of the Publisher to inadvertently disparage or overlook any individual, group, or entity.

It's important to underscore that, akin to any endeavor in life, especially those pertaining to health and fitness, there is no guarantee of monetary gain or specific outcomes from the advice dispensed in this book. Readers are therefore urged to apply their judgment and discretion, tailoring the guidance to fit their unique circumstances.

Moreover, this publication is not designed to be a substitute for professional advice in the realms of legal, business, accounting, or financial consulting. Readers are strongly encouraged to seek out and engage the expertise of professionals in these fields for guidance tailored to their specific needs.

Introduction

The story is all too common: embarking on a health and fitness journey filled with enthusiasm and possibly grand announcements, only to see that initial fervor wane and the plans fall by the wayside within a week. This pattern prompts a crucial reflection on why our commitment to diet plans, morning runs, and exercise regimes often falters. More importantly, it raises the question of how we can maintain these commitments, not just for our benefit but for those who depend on us.

This situation invites a deeper examination of our motivations for eating. Do we eat merely to quell hunger or to experience pleasure? Or do we see our dietary choices as a means to exert greater control over our lives?

This eBook delves into how conscious, deliberate food choices can significantly enhance our overall health and well-being. Through the adoption of regulated eating strategies, we aim to redefine our relationship with food, seeing it not as an adversary but as a valuable ally in our quest for a healthier, more rewarding life.

The path to a healthier lifestyle is strewn with obstacles and setbacks, not just of a physical nature but also psychological barriers that often undermine our resolve. Why is it that adherence to health and fitness commitments proves so challenging for many of us? A critical examination of the psychological factors at play

Chapter 1: Understanding Our Health and Fitness Challenges

Overview

In a time when health and fitness initiatives seem more likely to fail than succeed, it's crucial to question why these well-intentioned efforts often lead to disappointment. The reasons are complex and multifaceted, not merely a matter of ineffective programs or insufficient resources. Instead, they're deeply rooted in significant shifts in our lifestyle and dietary habits over recent decades, contributing to a world that seems increasingly unhealthy.

The Core Issue

The pervasive narrative of diet and fitness plan failures often overlooks a critical aspect: the onus of persistence and follow-through lies not with the programs but with the individuals who embark on them. Initial enthusiasm, frequently shared among peers and social circles, dwindles, leading to the premature abandonment of these health initiatives. This lack of commitment means the potential benefits of these programs go unrealized, inviting undue skepticism about their efficacy.

The Need for Motivation and Mindset

In addressing the health challenges of today,

what is needed is not necessarily an array of new health or fitness programs, but a profound shift in motivation and mindset. A significant transformation in the way we approach our health and fitness goals is crucial. This involves cultivating an inner drive and determination to adhere to the plans we set for ourselves, recognizing that the power to change resides within. If we can harness this motivation, many of the health issues stemming from lifestyle choices could be markedly reduced or even eliminated. This inner motivation is not something that requires searching far and wide; it lies within us, ready to be tapped into and utilized.

Reflecting on Dietary Choices

A mere generation ago, the concept of regularly consuming fast food as a staple diet was inconceivable. Today, it has become disturbingly common to equate hunger with a craving for fast food, often accompanied by sugary beverages and snacks. Modern dieting trends, too, tend towards seeking quick fixes that promise rapid weight loss but often neglect the importance of nutritional balance, leading to adverse health outcomes.

The Global Perspective

The challenge of improving public health extends beyond individual decisions; it's a global issue driven by collective dietary habits. The alarming rise in obesity rates in countries like the United States, with projections only suggesting further increases, underscores the urgency of addressing this issue. Yet, the concern is not solely about the individual choices we make; it's about the wider implications of these choices, including their environmental and societal impacts.

A Call to Action

This chapter encourages readers to reflect deeply on their health and lifestyle choices, highlighting the need for a disciplined approach to diet and fitness. It's crucial to understand that the success or failure of health programs often has more to do with our level of commitment than with the programs themselves. Embracing better health is not just a personal goal; it's a commitment to contributing positively to global health standards and making choices that benefit not just ourselves but the world around us.

As we move forward, it's important to remember that every health program, diet plan, or fitness routine holds the potential for success if approached with dedication and a willingness to commit fully. The true challenge lies not in finding the perfect plan but in finding within ourselves the resolve to pursue a healthier life, for our benefit and for the well-being of those around us.

Chapter 2: Shifting Your Mindset

Overview

The foundation of maintaining any health and fitness regime is not external—it doesn't lie in the hands of trainers or medical professionals, but within the realm of personal motivation and self-determination. The success of a health journey hinges on an individual's readiness to critically evaluate and adjust their lifestyle habits. Whether aiming to lose weight, enhance fitness levels, or manage health conditions, the commitment to adhere to a nutritious diet and consistent exercise routine is paramount.

Importance of Self-Determination

Recognizing that the path to better health requires more than just following professional advice is a crucial first step. It involves a comprehensive commitment to reshaping lifestyle choices. Losing weight, for example, transcends mere physical activity to encompass significant dietary changes. Similarly, managing a health condition isn't limited to medication adherence; it demands an overall lifestyle overhaul.

Rethinking Nutritional Choices

The dietary dilemma we face today is largely a product of a gradual departure from wholesome eating practices. To counteract this, a renewed emphasis on nutritional education is vital. Understanding which foods nourish our bodies and which detract from our health is the first step. This entails a shift towards a diet that includes fewer harmful substances like excess sugars, fats, and unnecessary carbohydrates, and more of the nutrients that bolster our health.

Challenging Conventional Wisdom

The diet industry's narrative, focused on dramatic transformations and quick fixes, often distracts from the sustainable path to health, which is based on mindful eating and regular physical activity. This industry-driven narrative overshadows the simple, yet profoundly effective steps individuals can take towards improving their health without resorting to expensive or restrictive diet plans.

The Path to a Healthier Diet

Contrary to popular belief, healthy eating does not mean sacrificing taste or enjoyment. There exists an abundance of nutritious foods that are as satisfying as they are beneficial. Discovering these alternatives and learning how to incorporate them into enjoyable meals can fundamentally change one's approach to dieting without feeling deprived.

Empowerment Through Knowledge and Action

While acknowledging the influence of the diet industry in shaping perceptions of health and nutrition, it's crucial to remember that the power for change lies within each individual. By educating ourselves about nutrition and committing to regular physical activity, we can reclaim control over our health. This empowerment doesn't necessitate reliance on commercial diet plans but rather encourages a personal commitment to understanding and caring for our bodies.

Commitment to Self and Others

Opting for a healthier lifestyle is ultimately an act of self-care and a declaration of respect for one's body. It's a commitment that extends beyond personal benefits to encompass the well-being of our families and communities. By choosing to adopt healthier habits, we not only improve our own lives but also contribute to a healthier society.

In this chapter, we delve into the necessity of a mindset shift—a move from seeking temporary fixes to embracing long-term, sustainable health practices. This commitment to health is not a solitary journey but a collective movement towards a healthier, more vibrant life for ourselves and those around us.

Chapter 3: The Many Benefits of Eating Right

Introduction

Embarking on a journey to eat right transcends mere diet modification; it's a commitment to transforming your entire lifestyle for the better. The benefits of adopting a nutritious diet are far-reaching, impacting not just personal health but also financial wellbeing and social life. This chapter explores the multitude of advantages associated with making informed and healthy dietary choices, providing ample motivation to pursue and maintain such a lifestyle change.

Health Improvements

The primary benefit of eating right is the profound impact it has on health. A diet rich in nutrients and balanced in its composition can significantly enhance metabolic functions, bolster the immune system, improve digestive health, and reduce the risk of many chronic diseases, including cardiovascular diseases, hypertension, and diabetes. The focus on whole, unprocessed foods over processed alternatives ensures that the body receives the essential nutrients it needs to function optimally, leading to improved overall health and vitality.

Economic Advantages

A common misconception is that eating healthily is more expensive than opting for processed or fast food options. However, a diet based on whole foods can actually lead to substantial savings. Reduced expenditure on processed foods, combined with lower healthcare costs resulting from improved health, can significantly lighten financial burdens. Additionally, mindful consumption encourages thoughtful purchasing habits, further enhancing financial wellbeing.

Reduced Intake of Toxins

In our industrialized food landscape, many products are laden with harmful chemicals and preservatives. By choosing natural, unprocessed foods, you drastically cut down the intake of these toxins. This shift not only contributes to better physical health but also often leads to reductions in unhealthy lifestyle choices, such as excessive alcohol consumption and smoking, as the body starts to crave more healthful sustenance.

Enhanced Physical and Social Life

Nutrition plays a critical role in energy levels and physical capability. A balanced diet fuels the body more effectively, enabling more active and fulfilling lifestyles. From increased physical endurance to enhanced ability to engage in social activities, the benefits of eating right extend far beyond the dinner plate. Moreover, as societal views often favor healthier body images, improving dietary habits can also lead to better social interactions and increased confidence.

Societal Perceptions and Personal Fulfillment

While societal norms unfairly judge individuals based on appearance and perceived self-discipline, adhering to a nutritious diet can positively influence how others perceive you. Beyond superficial benefits, making healthful dietary choices fosters a sense of personal achievement and fulfillment. Knowing that you are taking steps to improve your health and potentially extend your lifespan is profoundly rewarding.

Conclusion

The decision to eat healthily is a comprehensive commitment that promises a host of benefits, touching on every aspect of life. From tangible health improvements and financial savings to enhanced social life and personal fulfillment, the advantages of this commitment are undeniable. As you continue on this path, let the benefits outlined in this chapter serve as a constant source of motivation, reminding you of the value of your efforts. The journey towards a healthier lifestyle is a rewarding one, with each healthful choice paving the way to a better, more vibrant life.

Chapter 4: Navigating Healthy Eating

Introduction

In today's world, where diet fads and conflicting nutritional advice abound, establishing a sustainable, healthy eating pattern can seem daunting. Yet, the essence of healthy eating is not about strict dietary limitations or depriving yourself of the foods you love. Instead, it's about feeling great, having more energy, improving your outlook, and stabilizing your mood. This chapter provides a comprehensive guide to navigating the complexities of healthy eating, making informed choices that support long-term health and wellness.

Understanding Your Body's Needs

The first step in navigating healthy eating is understanding the unique needs of your body. This involves determining your daily caloric requirements based on your metabolism, physical activity level, and body composition. Recognizing that these needs can vary significantly from person to person is crucial. Tailoring your diet to meet these specific requirements ensures that you provide your body with the right amount of energy and nutrients.

The Importance of Healthy Fats

Fats have often been demonized in the dieting world, yet they are an essential component of a healthy diet. The key is to focus on consuming healthy fats, which can help to lower the risk of heart disease, improve brain function, and provide long-lasting energy. Sources of healthy fats include avocados, nuts, seeds, olive oil, and fatty fish like salmon. Integrating these into your diet can support overall health without contributing to weight gain.

Choosing the Right Carbohydrates

Carbohydrates are the body's primary energy source, but not all carbs are created equal. Opting for complex carbohydrates found in whole grains, vegetables, and fruits ensures a slower release of energy, helping to regulate blood sugar levels and keep you feeling full longer. Avoiding simple carbohydrates, such as those found in processed foods, sugary snacks, and white bread, can prevent energy spikes and crashes.

The Role of Protein

Protein is a critical building block of bones, muscles, cartilage, skin, and blood. Including a source of protein in every meal can help you maintain muscle mass, especially important as you age. Good sources of protein include lean meats, poultry, fish, beans, legumes, and dairy products. Plant-based proteins, such as quinoa and tofu, can also provide essential nutrients while offering variety in your diet.

Meal Timing and Portion Control

How and when you eat can be just as important as what you eat. Eating larger meals early in the day when your metabolism is more active, and reducing portion sizes in the evening can help manage weight and energy levels. Additionally, eating smaller, more frequent meals throughout the day can help keep your metabolism active and prevent overeating.

Hydration

Staying hydrated is an often-overlooked aspect of healthy eating. Water supports every metabolic function and nutrient transfer in the body and is essential for good health. Drinking adequate amounts of water can also aid in weight management by helping you feel full and reducing the likelihood of mistaking thirst for hunger.

Conclusion

Healthy eating is a journey that involves making informed choices about what, when, and how much to eat. By understanding your body's needs, choosing nutrient-rich foods, and adopting healthy eating habits, you can navigate the path to long-term health and wellness. Remember, the goal of healthy eating is not just to improve your physical appearance but to enrich your life in every aspect, providing the energy and vitality needed to pursue your passions and enjoy life to the fullest.

Chapter 5: Keeping Track of Progress

Introduction

Embarking on a journey towards healthier eating habits is a commendable endeavor that can significantly enhance your quality of life. However, to ensure that this journey yields lasting benefits, it's vital to monitor your progress. Keeping track not only helps in maintaining motivation but also in adjusting your strategy to better suit your needs as you move forward. This chapter discusses the importance of tracking your progress in healthy eating and how it can be a catalyst for sustained success.

The Motivational Power of Visible Progress

Humans are inherently motivated by progress and achievements. Seeing tangible results from your efforts in adopting healthier eating habits can be incredibly motivating. Whether it's noticing improvements in your physical health, such as weight loss or increased energy levels, or achieving milestones in your dietary goals, like reducing sugar intake, tracking these changes can reinforce your commitment to maintaining these new habits.

Tools and Techniques for Tracking

There are numerous methods for tracking progress in your healthy eating journey, ranging from traditional pen and paper to sophisticated digital apps. Food diaries, for instance, can help you become more mindful of your eating patterns, identify triggers for unhealthy eating, and recognize areas for improvement. Nutritional tracking apps can simplify the process by allowing you to log meals, monitor caloric intake, and understand your macronutrient distribution. These tools can offer insights into your nutritional habits and help tailor your diet to meet your specific health goals.

Setting Realistic and Measurable Goals

Effective progress tracking begins with setting realistic and measurable goals. Instead of vague objectives like "eat healthier," aim for specific targets such as "incorporate two servings of vegetables into every meal" or "drink 8 glasses of water daily." These clear, achievable goals make it easier to monitor your progress and celebrate victories along the way.

Reflecting and Adjusting Your Approach

Tracking your progress is not just about documenting successes; it's also about reflecting on the challenges and learning from them. Regularly reviewing your food diary or app data can help you identify patterns or behaviors that may hinder your progress. This reflection can guide necessary adjustments to your eating habits, ensuring that your approach to healthy eating evolves to meet your changing needs and preferences.

Celebrating Milestones

Every step towards healthier eating, no matter how small, deserves recognition. Celebrating milestones reinforces positive behavior and keeps you motivated. Whether it's treating yourself to a massage after a month of consistent healthy eating or simply acknowledging your efforts with a moment of gratitude, recognizing your achievements can boost your morale and commitment.

Conclusion

Keeping track of your progress in healthy eating is a crucial component of a successful wellness journey. It not only provides motivation but also offers valuable insights into your dietary habits, enabling you to make informed adjustments along the way. By setting realistic goals, utilizing tracking tools, reflecting on your journey, and celebrating your achievements, you can maintain momentum and continue to reap the benefits of a healthier lifestyle. Remember, the journey to better health is a marathon, not a sprint; every step forward, no matter how small, is a step in the right direction.

Chapter 6: Overcoming Challenges and Setbacks

Introduction

Transitioning to healthier eating habits is a commendable goal, but like any significant lifestyle change, it is often accompanied by its fair share of challenges and setbacks. From social pressures and environmental temptations to internal struggles such as cravings and old habits, various obstacles can derail even the most well-intentioned plans. However, overcoming these hurdles is not only possible but also a critical part of the journey towards sustained health and wellness. This chapter explores common challenges encountered on the path to healthier eating and strategies to overcome them, ensuring that setbacks become stepping stones rather than stumbling blocks.

Identifying Common Challenges

One of the first steps in overcoming obstacles is to identify them clearly. Common challenges include:

- **Cravings for Unhealthy Foods:** These are often triggered by stress, emotional discomfort, or habit.

- **Social and Environmental Pressures:** Social gatherings, workplace environments, or living situations can present temptations or pressures to indulge in less healthy eating habits.

- **Lack of Time and Convenience:** Busy schedules can make it tempting to opt for fast food or processed options instead of preparing nutritious meals.

- **Information Overload:** Conflicting dietary advice can lead to confusion and indecision about what healthy eating should look like.

Strategies for Overcoming Challenges

Once you've identified the specific challenges you face, you can employ targeted strategies to address them:

- **Plan Ahead:** Meal planning and preparation can help you resist the temptation to reach for unhealthy options when you're hungry and short on time.

- **Seek Support:** Surrounding yourself with a supportive community, whether online or in-person, can provide encouragement and accountability.

- **Manage Cravings:** Learning to distinguish between true hunger and emotional cravings can help you make healthier choices. Finding healthier alternatives that satisfy cravings without derailing your diet can also be effective.

- **Educate Yourself:** Gaining a solid understanding of nutrition can help you navigate conflicting advice and make informed decisions about your diet.

- **Set Realistic Expectations:** Recognizing that perfection is unattainable and that occasional indulgences are part of a balanced life can help prevent feelings of guilt or failure.

Embracing Setbacks as Learning Opportunities

Setbacks are an inevitable part of any change process, but they can also be invaluable learning opportunities. When you slip up, take the time to reflect on what led to the setback, what you could do differently next time, and how you can better prepare for similar challenges in the future. This reflective process can transform setbacks into powerful tools for growth and resilience.

Staying Flexible and Adaptable

A flexible, adaptable approach to healthy eating is more sustainable than rigid dietary rules. Life is unpredictable, and your eating habits need to be able to accommodate changes in your schedule, social life, and emotional state. Adopting a principle-based approach to nutrition rather than a prescriptive set of rules can help you maintain healthy eating habits in a variety of circumstances.

Conclusion

Overcoming the challenges associated with transitioning to healthier eating habits requires a combination of preparation, support, self-education, and self-compassion. By identifying common obstacles and employing targeted strategies to address them, you can navigate the path to healthier eating with confidence. Remember, setbacks are not failures but opportunities to learn and grow. With perseverance and a positive mindset, you can achieve and maintain a healthier, more fulfilling lifestyle.

Chapter 7: Integrating Healthy Eating into Your Lifestyle

Introduction

Adopting healthy eating habits is more than a temporary change; it's about integrating these practices into your daily life to create a sustainable lifestyle. This integration involves not just adjusting what you eat, but also how you think about food and its role in your life. It's about making healthy eating a seamless part of your day-to-day existence, one that complements your routines, preferences, and individual health goals. In this chapter, we explore strategies for making healthy eating an enduring component of your lifestyle, ensuring that it enhances your life rather than complicating it.

Creating a Supportive Environment

A conducive environment is key to sustaining healthy eating habits. This includes:

- **Stocking Healthy Options:** Ensure your pantry and refrigerator are filled with healthy, appealing options. Having nutritious foods readily available discourages the temptation to reach for less healthy snacks.

- **Designing a Healthy Kitchen Layout:** Arrange your kitchen so that healthier choices are the easiest to access. For example, place fruits and vegetables at eye level in the refrigerator.

- **Creating Meal Rituals:** Establishing regular meal times and places can help reinforce healthy eating habits. Making mealtime a special part of your day encourages mindfulness and enjoyment of food.

Incorporating Flexibility

Rigidity can be the enemy of sustainability. Incorporating flexibility into your approach to healthy eating can help you maintain your habits in the face of life's unpredictability. This means allowing yourself to enjoy treats in moderation, being adaptable with your meal choices when dining out or traveling, and not beating yourself up over occasional indulgences.

Making Informed Choices

Education is a powerful tool for sustaining healthy eating habits. Understanding the nutritional value of foods, how to read labels, and the basics of meal planning and preparation can empower you to make choices that align with your health goals. Continuous learning about nutrition and wellness can keep you motivated and informed.

Balancing Nutrition and Pleasure

Healthy eating should not be about deprivation but finding a balance between nutrition and enjoyment. This involves:

- **Exploring New Foods:** Experiment with different cuisines and ingredients to discover healthy foods that you enjoy.

- **Savoring Your Meals:** Eating slowly and mindfully can enhance the pleasure of eating and help prevent overeating.

- **Balancing Treats:** Find a healthy balance between enjoying your favorite treats and maintaining a nutritious diet.

Integrating Physical Activity

Physical activity complements healthy eating in promoting overall wellness. Finding forms of exercise that you enjoy and incorporating them into your routine can enhance the benefits of your healthy eating habits, improve mood, and boost energy levels.

Conclusion

Integrating healthy eating into your lifestyle is a journey that involves creating a supportive environment, embracing flexibility, making informed choices, balancing nutrition with pleasure, and complementing your diet with physical activity. By adopting a holistic approach to wellness, you can ensure that healthy eating becomes a natural and enjoyable part of your daily life. Remember, the goal is not just to live longer but to live better, with more vitality, joy, and health.

Chapter 8: Celebrating Your Healthy Eating Journey

Introduction

Embarking on a healthy eating journey is an accomplishment worth celebrating. It's a path that requires commitment, discipline, and a willingness to embrace change—qualities that contribute not only to better physical health but also to personal growth and self-awareness. As you progress on this journey, taking time to celebrate your achievements and reflect on the positive changes in your life is essential. This chapter focuses on recognizing your successes, embracing the transformative power of healthy eating, and looking forward to the continued benefits it brings to your life.

Acknowledging Milestones

Every step towards healthier eating, whether big or small, is a milestone that deserves recognition. Celebrating these achievements can range from acknowledging a week of balanced meals to commemorating a year of mindful eating. These milestones serve as reminders of your progress and commitment to your health. Consider keeping a journal or using an app to document these successes, giving you a tangible record of your journey.

The Transformative Power of Healthy Eating

Healthy eating has the potential to transform not just your physical health but your overall well-being. Reflect on the changes you've experienced since beginning your journey—improvements in energy levels, mood, sleep quality, and even mental clarity. These transformations are significant achievements that extend beyond the dinner plate, impacting every area of your life.

Sharing Your Journey

Sharing your journey with others can be a powerful way to celebrate your progress. Whether it's through social media, a blog, or conversations with friends and family, talking about your experiences can inspire others and create a sense of community. Sharing your story can also reinforce your commitment to healthy eating and provide motivation to continue on this path.

Continuing Education and Experimentation

A commitment to healthy eating is also a commitment to continuous learning and exploration. Celebrate your journey by seeking out new knowledge about nutrition, experimenting with different foods and recipes, and even attending workshops or cooking classes. This approach keeps the journey exciting and ensures that your healthy eating habits never feel stagnant or monotonous.

Setting New Goals

As you achieve your initial health and nutrition goals, set new ones to keep yourself challenged and engaged. These goals can be related to trying new foods, mastering specific cooking techniques, or even improving other areas of health and wellness, such as physical fitness or stress management. Setting and achieving new goals is a vital part of keeping your healthy eating journey dynamic and rewarding.

Conclusion

Celebrating your healthy eating journey is about more than just acknowledging your dietary changes; it's about recognizing the profound impact these changes have on your life. It's a celebration of the hard work, learning, and personal growth that comes with committing to a healthier lifestyle. By acknowledging milestones, embracing the transformative power of healthy eating, sharing your journey, continuing to learn, and setting new goals, you ensure that your journey is not just sustainable but also deeply fulfilling. Here's to celebrating every step of your journey towards a healthier, happier you.

Chapter 9: Nurturing a Community of Healthy Eaters

Introduction

As you journey further into the realm of healthy eating, one transformative realization often emerges: the journey is richer and more impactful when shared. Nurturing a community of like-minded individuals who prioritize healthful eating can amplify your own experiences, providing a network of support, inspiration, and collective wisdom. This chapter delves into the importance of building and engaging with a community of healthy eaters, offering strategies for creating meaningful connections that foster mutual growth and encouragement in the pursuit of wellness.

The Power of Shared Goals

Embarking on a path towards healthier eating habits can sometimes feel isolating, especially if those in your immediate social circles do not share your enthusiasm or goals. However, connecting with others who are on similar journeys can provide a sense of belonging and understanding that is profoundly motivating. Whether it's celebrating victories, sharing struggles, or exchanging tips, the communal aspect of shared goals creates a powerful synergy that can propel each member forward.

Creating Your Community

Building a community of healthy eaters can begin in your own backyard or extend globally, thanks to digital platforms. Here are some avenues to explore:

- **Local Meetups and Cooking Classes:** Participating in or organizing local meetups focused on healthy eating or cooking classes can foster face-to-face connections with others who share your interests.

- **Online Forums and Social Media:** Joining online communities and social media groups focused on healthy eating provides access to a vast network of individuals from diverse backgrounds, offering varying perspectives and insights.

- **Workplace Initiatives:** Initiating or participating in health and wellness programs at your workplace can help cultivate a culture of healthy eating among colleagues.

Engaging and Contributing

Active participation and contribution are key to nurturing a thriving community. Sharing your experiences, successes, and challenges not only helps others but also reinforces your commitment to your health goals. Engaging in meaningful discussions, offering support, and providing constructive feedback create a dynamic environment where everyone can learn and grow.

Organizing Community Events

Organizing events such as potlucks, recipe swaps, or group challenges can add a fun and interactive dimension to your community. These gatherings serve as opportunities to bond over shared interests, celebrate progress, and enjoy the collective journey towards better health.

Leveraging Community Knowledge

A community of healthy eaters is a treasure trove of knowledge and experience. From discovering new recipes to learning about nutrition, the collective wisdom of the community can be an invaluable resource. Encourage knowledge sharing through workshops, guest speakers, or collaborative content creation to enrich the community's understanding and practice of healthy eating.

Conclusion

Fostering a community of healthy eaters is not just about enhancing your own journey towards wellness; it's about contributing to a larger movement that values health, nutrition, and mutual support. By connecting with others, sharing experiences, and learning together, you create a vibrant network that celebrates the joys and navigates the challenges of healthy eating. In this community, each member finds not only encouragement and motivation but also the joy of contributing to the collective well-being and growth. Together, you move forward, enriching not just your meals but also your lives with the essence of healthful camaraderie.

Chapter 10: The Future of Healthy Eating

Introduction

As we look towards the future, the landscape of healthy eating is poised for transformative shifts influenced by technological advancements, environmental considerations, and a deeper understanding of human nutrition. This evolving scenario presents both opportunities and challenges for individuals committed to a lifestyle of healthful eating. Embracing these changes and preparing for what lies ahead can ensure that your journey towards wellness remains dynamic, informed, and aligned with broader global trends.

Technological Innovations and Personalized Nutrition

The future of healthy eating is intricately linked with advancements in technology. From apps that track nutritional intake in real-time to genetic testing that offers personalized dietary recommendations, technology is set to revolutionize how we approach nutrition. Embracing these tools can enhance your ability to make informed decisions about your diet, tailor your eating habits to your body's unique needs, and navigate the complexities of nutritional science with greater ease.

Sustainability and Ethical Eating

An increasing awareness of the environmental impact of our food choices is driving a shift towards more sustainable and ethically sourced diets. This includes a greater emphasis on plant-based eating, locally sourced produce, and practices that reduce food waste. Integrating these considerations into your healthy eating habits not only contributes to your well-being but also supports the health of the planet.

The Role of Community in Shaping Dietary Trends

As you've nurtured a community of healthy eaters, it's important to recognize the collective power such communities have in shaping future dietary trends. By advocating for healthier, more sustainable food options and supporting ethical food production practices, communities can influence the food industry, policy-making, and public health initiatives, driving positive change on a larger scale.

Adapting to Global Dietary Changes

Globalization and cultural exchange are enriching the world's culinary landscape, introducing a plethora of new foods, flavors, and nutrition philosophies. Staying open to these influences can broaden your dietary horizons, enrich your palette, and provide a more diverse array of nutrients to your diet. Embracing global dietary changes can also foster a greater sense of connection and appreciation for the world's cultures and their approaches to health and nutrition.

Continued Learning and Adaptation

The field of nutrition is constantly evolving, with new research shedding light on the complex relationship between diet, health, and disease. Staying informed about the latest scientific discoveries and nutritional guidelines is crucial for adapting your eating habits to the latest evidence-based recommendations. Continued education and a willingness to revise your approach in light of new information will be key to navigating the future of healthy eating successfully.

Conclusion

The future of healthy eating is bright, characterized by advancements that promise greater personalization, an emphasis on sustainability, and a global palette of nutritional options. As you move forward, let your journey be guided by a spirit of curiosity, adaptability, and a commitment to not just your health, but the well-being of the planet and its inhabitants. By embracing change, advocating for positive shifts in the food system, and continuously seeking knowledge, you can play an active role in shaping a future where healthy eating is accessible, enjoyable, and beneficial for all.

With the journey through the foundational elements of embracing a healthier lifestyle and the nuances of nurturing a sustainable, healthful eating habit concluding, the road ahead is ripe with the promise of personal growth, community engagement, and a deeper connection with the very essence of nourishment. The chapters of this guide have equipped you with knowledge, strategies, and a philosophical outlook on the transformative power of mindful eating. Yet, as we venture beyond the pages of this book, the narrative of your wellness odyssey continues to unfold in the daily choices you make and the moments of insight you gain. Here's a glimpse into the unwritten chapters that await your exploration.

Exploring the Horizon of Holistic Health

Healthful eating is a vital component of wellness, but it's just one piece of a larger puzzle. The journey ahead invites you to explore holistic health practices that complement your nutritional choices. This exploration could lead you to delve into physical activity routines that resonate with your body's needs, mindfulness practices to enhance mental well-being, and restorative sleep habits to recharge your spirit.

Innovating Your Nutritional Journey

As science advances and our understanding of nutrition deepens, new opportunities to innovate your dietary practices will emerge. Stay curious and open to experimenting with emerging superfoods, alternative dietary patterns, and cutting-edge nutritional science. This continuous innovation will not only sustain your interest in healthful eating but also enable you to adapt to the evolving landscape of wellness.

Building Bridges Through Culinary Diversity

Food is a universal language that transcends cultural barriers, and your journey ahead is an invitation to build bridges through the exploration of culinary diversity. Engaging with different cultures through their food can enrich your palate, broaden your nutritional intake, and deepen your appreciation for the global tapestry of culinary traditions. This exploration is an opportunity to celebrate diversity, learn from various health philosophies, and integrate global wisdom into your wellness practice.

Advancing Sustainability in Your Food Choices

The future of healthful eating is inextricably linked to the sustainability of our food systems. As you move forward, consider how your food choices impact the environment and what steps you can take to promote sustainability. This might involve supporting local and organic farmers, reducing food waste, and advocating for food policies that prioritize the health of the planet alongside human nutrition.

Empowering Others on Their Wellness Paths

Your journey has the power to inspire and empower others. Sharing your experiences, insights, and lessons learned can light the way for those just beginning their path to wellness. Whether through mentorship, community initiatives, or simply leading by example, your journey can contribute to a collective shift towards a more health-conscious and sustainable society.

Conclusion

The chapters ahead are unwritten, inviting your pen to script a future where healthful eating and holistic wellness are not just aspirations but lived realities. Your journey is both personal and universal, a single thread woven into the larger fabric of our collective quest for health and vitality. As you continue to navigate the complexities and joys of this path, remember that every step taken with intention is a step towards a healthier, more vibrant you and a more sustainable world. Let the journey continue.

With the path ahead rich in potential and the canvas of your wellness journey vast and waiting for your brush, it's essential to anchor in the understanding that this is not merely an end but a beginning. A beginning of deeper exploration into wellness, a sustained commitment to nurturing your body and mind, and a continuous embrace of the community and environment around you. As we step beyond the structured chapters of guidance and advice, we venture into the realm of lifelong learning and growth, where the principles of healthy eating intertwine with the broader tapestry of living a balanced, fulfilled life.

Embracing Lifelong Wellness

Your journey toward healthier eating habits is a cornerstone of a broader pursuit of lifelong wellness. This ongoing quest encompasses not only what you eat but also how you live, think, and interact with the world around you. Embracing wellness in its entirety involves nurturing your physical health, cultivating mental and emotional resilience, fostering meaningful relationships, and pursuing activities that bring joy and fulfilment.

The Evolution of Personal and Collective Well-being

As you continue to evolve on your journey, remember that personal well-being and collective health are deeply interconnected. Your choices, from the foods you eat to the products you consume, have ripple effects on the health of communities, economies, and the planet. Moving forward, consider how you can contribute to a more sustainable, equitable, and health-conscious world through your everyday decisions and actions.

Continued Growth and Adaptation

The landscape of nutrition and wellness is ever-changing, with new research, trends, and technologies continuously emerging. Staying informed, open-minded, and adaptable will allow you to navigate these changes effectively, integrating new knowledge into your lifestyle in ways that enhance your health and well-being. Seek out reputable sources of information, engage with experts and communities, and be willing to adjust your approach as you learn and grow.

Fostering Community and Connection

The strength of the community has been a recurring theme in your journey toward healthier eating. As you move forward, continue to build and nurture connections with those who share your values and aspirations. Whether through local initiatives, online platforms, or personal relationships, these connections can provide support, inspiration, and a sense of belonging. Together, you can celebrate successes, navigate challenges, and drive positive change.

The Journey Is Yours

As we conclude this guide, it's clear that the journey of healthy eating and overall wellness is deeply personal and uniquely yours. It's a journey marked by discovery, growth, and moments of both challenge and triumph. Embrace this journey with compassion for yourself and others, a commitment to lifelong learning, and a vision for the positive impact you can make in the world.

Remember, each step you take on this path is a reflection of your dedication to living your best life—a life of vitality, purpose, and harmony with yourself and the world around you. Here's to the journey ahead, filled with health, happiness, and endless possibilities.

As we close this comprehensive guide on transforming your relationship with food and embracing a lifestyle of healthful eating, it's clear that the journey doesn't end here. The path to wellness is ongoing, a continuous cycle of learning, growing, and adapting to new knowledge, experiences, and the changing world around us. While this book has provided you with the tools, insights, and encouragement to embark on and sustain this journey, the future chapters of your wellness story are yours to write.

Living a Life Enriched by Healthy Eating

The principles of healthy eating, once integrated into your daily life, have the power to enrich not just your physical health but your overall sense of well-being. As you move forward, remember that healthful eating is not just about the food on your plate but about nurturing your body, mind, and spirit. It's about making choices that reflect your values, enhance your life, and contribute to the world around you.

Embracing Change with Confidence

The world of nutrition and wellness will continue to evolve, bringing new challenges and opportunities. Facing these changes with confidence requires an open mind and a commitment to continued learning. Whether it's adapting to new dietary guidelines, incorporating emerging superfoods into your meals, or finding innovative ways to stay active, approach these changes as opportunities to enhance your journey towards health and vitality.

Advocating for Health and Sustainability

As a member of the global community of healthy eaters, you have a voice in the conversation about food, health, and sustainability. Use this voice to advocate for changes that promote the availability of nutritious, ethically produced food for everyone. Supporting local farmers, choosing sustainable food options, and encouraging policies that promote health and environmental stewardship are ways you can make a difference.

Fostering Wellness in Your Community

The journey towards healthful eating and wellness is more rewarding when shared. Continue to build and nurture your community of healthy eaters, sharing your knowledge, experiences, and support with others. Whether through organizing local wellness events, leading healthy cooking workshops, or simply sharing a meal with friends, you can inspire and uplift those around you on their own paths to wellness.

The Next Steps on Your Journey

As you look to the future, consider the next steps on your journey. Set new goals, explore new foods and cultures, and challenge yourself to grow in areas of wellness that you have yet to explore. Remember, the journey to healthful eating is not linear; it's a rich tapestry of experiences that shape you, teach you, and allow you to live your fullest life.

Closing Thoughts

Thank you for embarking on this journey through the world of healthful eating and wellness. As you continue to explore, experiment, and evolve on your path, keep in mind that every choice you make has the power to transform your health and the world around you. Here's to a future filled with vibrant health, profound wellness, and joyous eating.

Table of contents for the guide:

- **Terms and Conditions & Legal Disclaimer**: Page 1

- **Introduction**: Page 2

- **Chapter 1: Understanding Our Health and Fitness Challenges**: Page 5

- **Chapter 2: Shifting Your Mindset**: Page 10

- **Chapter 3: The Many Benefits of Eating Right**: Page 15

- **Chapter 4: Navigating Healthy Eating**: Page 20

- **Chapter 5: Keeping Track of Progress**: Page 25

- **Chapter 6: Overcoming Challenges and Setbacks**: Page 30

- **Chapter 7: Integrating Healthy Eating into Your Lifestyle**: Page 35

- **Chapter 8: Celebrating Your Healthy Eating Journey**: Page 40

- **Chapter 9: Nurturing a Community of Healthy Eaters**: Page 45

- **Chapter 10: The Future of Healthy Eating**: Page 50

- **Epilogue**: Page 55